YOUR KNOWLEDGE HAS VALUE

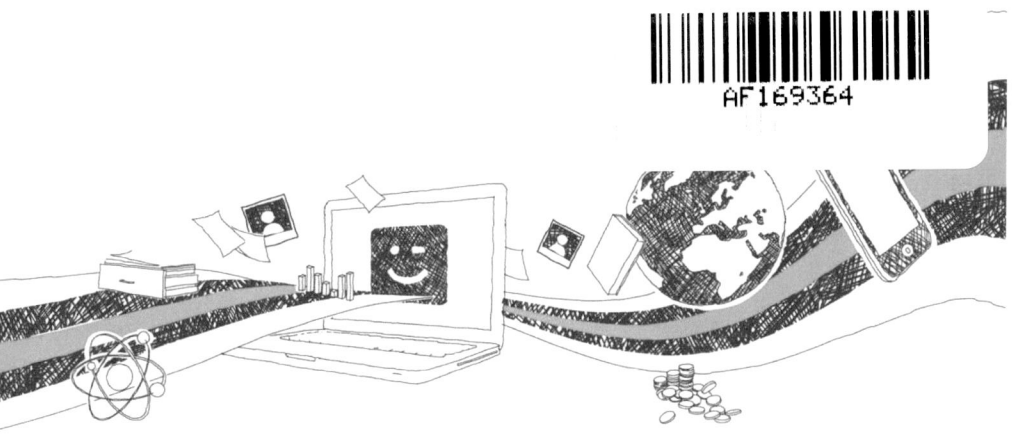

- We will publish your bachelor's and master's thesis, essays and papers

- Your own eBook and book - sold worldwide in all relevant shops

- Earn money with each sale

Upload your text at www.GRIN.com and publish for free

Bibliographic information published by the German National Library:

The German National Library lists this publication in the National Bibliography; detailed bibliographic data are available on the Internet at http://dnb.dnb.de .

This book is copyright material and must not be copied, reproduced, transferred, distributed, leased, licensed or publicly performed or used in any way except as specifically permitted in writing by the publishers, as allowed under the terms and conditions under which it was purchased or as strictly permitted by applicable copyright law. Any unauthorized distribution or use of this text may be a direct infringement of the author s and publisher s rights and those responsible may be liable in law accordingly.

Imprint:

Copyright © 2016 GRIN Verlag, Open Publishing GmbH
Print and binding: Books on Demand GmbH, Norderstedt Germany
ISBN: 9783668575516

This book at GRIN:

http://www.grin.com/en/e-book/381306/food-bioprocessing-solid-state-fermentation

Patrick Kimuyu

Food Bioprocessing. Solid State Fermentation

GRIN Publishing

GRIN - Your knowledge has value

Since its foundation in 1998, GRIN has specialized in publishing academic texts by students, college teachers and other academics as e-book and printed book. The website www.grin.com is an ideal platform for presenting term papers, final papers, scientific essays, dissertations and specialist books.

Visit us on the internet:

http://www.grin.com/

http://www.facebook.com/grincom

http://www.twitter.com/grin_com

Food Bioprocessing: Solid State Fermentation

Name: Patrick K. Kimuyu

The Table of Contents

1.0 Introduction 3
1.1 Substrates used in Solid-State Fermentation 3
1.2 Microorganisms in SSF 4
1.3 Bioreactors in SSF 6
1.4 Biochemical Engineering Principles Applied in Solid State Fermentation 6
1.5 Applications of Solid-State Fermentations 9
1.6 Conclusion 12
References 13

1.0 Introduction

For centuries, fermentation has been extensively applied in the production of distinct substances that remain highly beneficial to industries and people, with its increasing techniques gaining immense significance due to their environmental and economic benefits. According to recent studies, solid state fermentation is considered as the cheapest and environmentally responsive approach for the production of value-added industrial products, for example, enzymes biofuels and even nutrient enriched animal feeds. Solid state fermentation may be described as the growth and/or cultivation of micro-organisms under controlled conditions without the presence of free liquid for desired products development. It is an ancient technique that utilizes solid substrates such as bagasse, paper pulp and bran. A key benefit of using such substrates is that waste substances that are rich in nutrients can be recycled as substrates, and due to the slow and steady substrate utilization, the substrate may be used for long fermentation periods. As a result, this technique sustains controlled nutrients release.

Significantly, solid-state fermentation technique works best in techniques that involve fungi as well as micro-organisms requiring less moisture content since the moisture required for the growth of microbes exists in absorbed states or in composite with solid matrix. However, even though this technique has diverse advantages, especially compared with submerged fermentation technique, there are certain processes in which SSF may not be used, for example, in bacterial fermentation or in processes that involve organisms requiring high water activity. The main aim of this paper is, thus, describing solid-state fermentation as a technique for the production of bioactive compounds.

1.1 Substrates used in Solid-State Fermentation

Notably, the result of fermentation shows a discrepancy in each substrate used; thus, it remains highly significant to select the right substrate, and fermentation techniques need to be optimized for every substrate since organisms react differently to the substrate. In addition, the utilization rates of distinct nutrients vary in each substrate, similar to the productivity level. With respect to SSF processes, several agro-industrial residues can be used as solid substrates, with the selection of these wastes depending on certain physical parameters, for example, the moisture level, particle size, intra-particle spacing alongside the substrate's nutrient composition (Bhargav *et al.*

2008). The main and common substrates that are used in solid-state fermentation include wheat bran, sugarcane and cassava bagasse, paper pulp, coconut coir and even synthetic media (Subramaniyam & Vimala, 2012). Other substrates that can also be used include coffee husks, orange bagasse, oil cakes, wheat and rice straws and even grape seeds and juice. Remarkably, cassava as well as sugarcane bagasse have been noted to have higher benefits compared to other substrates like wheat and rice straws since they contain low ash content. In this sense, cassava is regarded as the optimal SSF substrate because it has a high capacity of retaining water (Bhargav *et al.* 2008). Furthermore, cassava bagasse is more preferred than sugarcane bagasse since it does not need pre-treatment and can easily be decomposed by several micro-organisms for distinct purposes. Cassava bagasse is extensively used in the production of citric acid, mushrooms, and different forms of flavours alongside being used in copious biotransformation processes. Conversely, wheat bran and sugarcane bagasse are utilized in commercial production of the majority of compounds using solid-state fermentation techniques. There are diverse economical applications associated with sugarcane bagasse including the production of cattle feeds enriched with proteins, and pre-treatment remains significant because of easy micro-organisms assimilation that results in hemicellulose and lignin decomposition. Coffee pulp or husk remains to be another rapid emerging agroindustrial substrate because it has high nutritive value and is rich in organic, although coffee husks are prone to fungi *Basidiomycetes* (Bhargav *et al.* 2008).

1.2 Microorganisms in SSF

Research exhibits that fungi, bacteria and yeast can grow on solid substrates and that they can find their application in solid-state fermentation. According to scholars, filamentous fungi remain to be the most adapted for this technique, with bacteria observed to be mainly engaged in composting, ensiling besides other food processes. Yeasts assume a critical portion in the production of ethanol and feed or food production. Filamentous fungi are the mostly preferred micro-organisms used in SSF process because of their biochemical, enzymological and physiological properties. The hyphae fungal growth mode and tolerance to low water quality, alongside high osmotic pressure conditions play significant roles in making fungi proficient and competitive in natural microflora for solid substrates bioconversion (Mienda *et al.* 2011). Auspiciously, *Koji* and *Tempeh* remain to be the major SSF applications with filamentous fungi. It is worth noting that the hyphal growth mode gives a significant advantage to fungi over unicellular micro-organisms in solid substrates colonization and for available nutrients utilization.

Table 1. Main Groups of micro-organisms involved in SSF (Mienda *et al.* 2011, p. 23)

Microflora	SSF Process
Bacteria	
Clostidrium sp.	Ensiling, Food
Lactobacillus sp.	Ensiling, Food
Streptoccus sp	Composting
Pseudomonas sp.	Composting
Serratia sp.	Composting
Bacillus sp.	Composting, Natto, amylase
Fungi	
Altemaria sp.	Composting
Penicilium notatum, roquefortii	Penicillin, Cheese
Lentinus edodes	Shii-take mushroom
Pleurotus oestreatus, sajor-caju	Mushroom
Aspergillus niger	Feed, Proteins, Amylase, citric acid
Rhizopus oligosporus	Tempeh, soybean, amylase, lipase
Aspergillus oryzae	Koji, Food, citric acid
Rhizopus sp.	Composting. Food, enzymes, organic acids
Aspergillus sp.	Composting, Industrial, Food
Yeast	
Endomicopsis burtonii	Tape, cassava, rice
Schwanniomyces castelli	Ethanol, Amylase

1.3 Bioreactors in SSF

The purpose of bioreactor systems in fermentation processes is to provide a conducive environment for microbial growth and/or cultivation. Nonetheless, the product's growth in SSF bioreactors is determined by several factors including temperature, the type of substrate used, substrate's bed humidity, bioreactor size, cooling rate, aeration along with the bed's height and fungal morphology (Bhargav *et al.* 2008, p. 54). SSF bioreactors are categorized into two groups; small-scale bioreactors and large-scale. In small-scale bioreactors, solid-state fermentation is performed in jars, Petri dishes, roux bottles, wide-mouthed Erlenmeyer flasks and roller bottles, characterized by simple systems and experiments that are done easily. Accordingly, there are numerous types of small-scale bioreactors, an example being column bioreactors that are made of small columns capable of holding twenty grams of pre-inoculated solid substance. Column bioreactors remain highly beneficial in medium optimization, although they pose a challenge in the product obtaining alongside heat removal. Another small-scale bioreactor is the INRA bioreactors that are highly advanced, and have been noted to have easier analysis sampling compared to ORSTOM bioreactors, all having automatic control of temperature and humidity (Bhargav *et al.* 2008). Again, there are other bioreactor systems with agitator systems apart from these non-agitated column reactors including horizontal paddle mixer and perforated-drum reactor. Advancements on these rotating drum bioreactors gave birth to Zymotis packed bed reactors and Growtek bioreactors.

In terms of large-scale bioreactors, the successful operation depends on the features gotten after mathematical modeling, substrate's susceptibility alongside fungal morphology in increasing temperature, particle size, substrate quantity and height of substrate bed. Some of the large-scale bioreactors used in SSF include the Koji reactors, PLAFRACTOR and rotating drum bioreactor (RDB) (Bhargav *et al.* 2008).

1.4 Biochemical Engineering Principles Applied in Solid State Fermentation

In the recent years, substantial studies have been carried out to understand SSF's engineering aspects such as in moisture and water activity in SSF, temperature and heat transfer, biomass and growth kinetics, mass transfer and modelling.

1.4.1 Moisture and Water Activity in SSF

Water activity (A_w) remains to be an extremely beneficial parameter for water potential measurement, typifying the energetic state of water. Water relations studies in SSF have been carried out under quantitative aspects. Evidently, the substrate's water activity highly influences microbial activity. The type of organisms that can develop in SSF is determined by A_w, whereby the medium's A_W remains to be a fundamental parameter for mass water transfer in the microbial cells. Therefore, this parameter's control may be used in the modification of microbial production and excretion (Bhargav *et al.* 2008). According to research, mycelia's radial extension rate, fungal spore production, secondary metabolites production and biomass production are all related or influenced by water activity.

1.4.2 Temperature and Heat Transfer

Temperatures, as well as heat transfer processes in the substrate's bed, have been noted to stimulate fungal growth alongside secondary metabolite production in SSF. In SSF, a significant amount of heat that is proportional to the micro-organism's metabolic activities is generated, although fungus can grow over a broad range of temperatures. The in and out transfer of heat of an SSF system is closely related with microbial metabolic activity alongside fermentation system's aeration. Additionally, high temperature is noted to affect fungal germination, formation of metabolites and even sporulation. Temperature and moisture control remains to be an issue of concern since poor thermal conductivity along with low moisture of the substrate makes this control intricate in SSF (Bhargav *et al.* 2008, p. 51).

1.4.3 Biomass and Growth Kinetics

Different scholars have demonstrated that biomass is a basic parameter in fungal growth characterization and is vital growth kinetics measurement in SSF. Conversely, it has been realized that culturing fungus over the membrane filter may perform direct biomass estimation since this membrane filter inhibits fungal hyphae penetration within the substrate. There are numerous methods that can be used in estimating fungal biomass in an SSF system such as electron microscope scanning, fungal biomass reaction with certain fluorochrome probes, and reflectance infrared (IR) spectroscopy. Again, this determination can be performed through biochemical methods, facilitated by the three constituents; Ergosterol, Glucosamine and total sugar (Bhargav et al. 2008).

1.4.4 Mass Transfer

In SSF, the gradients of inter-particle concentration rising from nutrient consumption together with mass transfer restrictions may constitute a strong impact on the process' rate and efficiency. There are two phenomena of mass transfer in SSF; micro-scale and macro-scale whereby micro-scale mass transfer is determined by the micro-organism's growth, which depends on oxygen and carbon dioxide intra- and inter-particles diffusion, nutrient absorption, enzymes and formation of metabolites (Bhargav et al. 2008, p. 51). On the other hand, micro-scale mass transfer involves the SSF's in and out airflow, substrate type, bioreactor design, substrate mixing, particles spacing, particle size variation and the micro-organisms present.

1.4.5 Modelling

Arguably, one of the major tools for optimal bioreactors design and operation remains to be the mathematical modelling in an SSF system. In this sense, the procured costs in projecting fermentation conditions in large-scale production are reduced. There are two distinctive types of bioreactor models: Kinetic and Transport models (Bhargav et al. 2008). In kinetic model, the manner by which micro-organisms are influenced by varied process parameters is described while in transport model, mass and heat transfer in the bioreactor SSF systems is described. The kinetic model is determined by the size of particles, packing density, substrate particles pore size, respiration rate, the fungal mycelium penetration depth in the substrate alongside the substrate's bed water content. On the other hand, transport model is determined by the fungus growth rate, the airflow rate through the bed, bed's height, and bioreactor walls width as well as heat removal process rate. In addition, these mathematical models aid in depicting the correlation between oxygen and the rate of substrate consumption, substrate consumption rate and that of biomass synthesis, biomass synthesis rate and that of oxygen uptake, alongside the biomass synthesis rate and heat evolved (Bhargav et al. 2008). Consequently, simulation and modelling of biological processes form an economic and ecological basis that facilitates integrated optimization of the SSF processes.

1.5 Applications of Solid-State Fermentations

1.5.1 Enzymes Production by SSF

One of the most crucial SSF applications remains to be enzyme production. SSF is renowned to consist of numerous advantages compared with submerged fermentation, for example; it has high volumetric productivity, better product yield, low equipment cost, less waste generation and less time consumption. Some of the enzymes produced include protease, lipase, cellulose, pectinase, phytase, L-glutaminase, amylase, ligninase and xylanase (Bhargav *et al.* 2008). As aforementioned, SSF is widely preferred in situations where enzymes have to be extracted from fungi that do not require high water potential. Notably, most of the enzymes produced in SSF system are derived from the fungi belonging to the genus *Aspergillus*, whereby its renowned benefits have granted it the opportunity of being a model organism for fungal enzyme production (Subramaniyam & Vimala, 2012,). Indeed, *A. niger* remains to be the single largest fungal source of enzymes.

Table 2. Enzyme Production by *Aspergillus* species (Subramaniyam & Vimala, 2012, 481)

Enzyme	Micro-organism	SSF Substrate	Productivity
Estrase	*Aspergillus niger*	sugar beet pulp	20 nkat/mg
Cellulose	*Trichoderma viride*	Wheat bran	60.5 nkat/mg
Invertase	*A. nigger (mutant)*	Polyurethane Foam	Higher
Lipase	*A. nigger*	Wheat bran & olive oil	630 IU/g
Phytase	*A. nigger*	wheat bran & soybean	884 U/g
Tannase	*A. nigger* Aa-20	Polyurethane foam	12, 000 IU/l

1.5.2 Production of Organic Acids under SSF

Fermentation techniques highly contribute in the production of organic acids, for instance, citric acid, fumaric acid, lactic acid, gallic acid, kojic acid and *y*-linoleic acid (Bhargav et al. 2008). The development and progress of producing organic acids remained sequential with the development of solid-state fermentation. Nevertheless, the biotechnological processes that are used in large-scale production of organic acids still lag in terms of development. Organic acids present high-profile economic benefits as they are the most common food and beverages ingredients worldwide. The main reason for this aspect is that they contain three critical properties namely, solubility, contain a hygroscopic ability alongside the ability to chelate (Bhargav *et al.* 2008).

1.5.3 Production of Antibiotics

Antibiotics represent the most crucial category of bioactive compounds that are extracted from micro-organisms by fermentation processes. Significantly, penicillin remains to be the first commercially extracted antibiotic using fermentation, which was carried out as early as 1940s by the use of SSF. Currently, several antibiotics have been produced through this technique, for example, cyclosporins, surfactins, cephalosporin, tetracyclins as well as streptomycin. In the past, nearly all of the production methods relied on submerged fermentation technique, but the development of appropriate substrates has resulted in widespread use of SSF (Subramaniyam & Vimala, 2012).

1.5.4 Production of Poly Gamma Glutamate (PGG)

Poly gamma glutamate refers to an anionic, water-soluble and a highly viscous form of polypeptides. It can be used as a thickener, drug carrier, humectants, feed additive and even as a heavy metal absorber. The limitation of oxygen along with mass transfer and unmanageable foaming is noted to decrease PGG production in submerged fermentation technique, but in SSF, foaming control and substrate's cost is attained. A noteworthy PGG production substrate using Bacillus subtilis is a high protein-containing substance; thus, wheat bran supplemented with soybean cake powder alongside additives like glutamate as substrate will result in maximal PGG production (Bhargav et al. 2008).

1.5.5 Production of Poly Unsaturated Fatty Acids

Polyunsaturated acids are not produced in the body, and; hence, they have to be supplied in the diet. Solid-state fermentation can be utilized in the production of these fatty acids. With respect to this, the fungus involved in the production of these fatty acids reduces anti-nutrient substances (for example, phytic acid) in the substrate, partially hydrolyzing the biopolymers in the substrate, thus, making them apt for food supplement (Bhargav et al. 2008). Mass transfer during fermentation remains to be the most important parameter to be considered in solid-state fermentation, together with the problems involved in scaling-up.

1.5.6 Poly Hydroxy Alkanoates

Poly hydroxy alkanoates refer to microbial polyesters that are accumulated by microbes for reserving energy. Radically, the production of these alkanoates by solid-state fermentation has been noted to reduce environmental challenges along with reducing the costs involved in the process (Bhargav et al. 2008). Several substrates, for example, olive oil, babassu oil cake that is treated with Rastonia eutropha may be utilized in producing poly hydroxy alkanoates using SSF. Moreover, including sugarcane molasses in soy cake elevates the production of these alkanoates.

1.5.7 Biofuel Production Using SSF

Nowadays, ethanol is regarded as the most widely used biofuel in different regions of the globe. SSF technique is substantially preferred in the production of ethanol, even though it is easier to produce it using the submerged fermentation technique. The main factors for this preference of the SSF technique include the lower water requirement, the ability to prevent inhibition of end product, small volumes of fermentation mash, along with the ability of discharging less liquid water, hence, decrease in pollution (Bhargav et al. 2008).

1.6 Conclusion

Evidently, the last two decades have witnessed an incessant and fast growth in solid-state fermentation technology. Although this technology may have some disadvantages, it is obvious that these challenges are outweighed by the copious benefits because of the fermentation engineering problems. In most of the SSF systems today, fungi are adequately suitable compared to bacterial and yeast strains, though if these two are genetically modified or engineered, they can suite in SSF. In order to curb the perceived challenges in SSF, extensive focus has to be directed on the problems in scale-up, heat generation and varied fermentation conditions, and on the unavailability of direct analytical processes in direct biomass determination in the substrate bed. Again, so as to produce high value added products, the bioreactors have to be improved alongside maintaining a process control for unremitting SSF. A crucial part of this process is maintaining proper substrate and additives optimization.

References

Bhargav, S., Panda, B. P., Ali, M., & Javed, S. (2008). Solid-state Fermentation: An Overview: *Chem. Biochem. Eng.*, 22(*1*), 49-70.

Mienda, B. S., Idi, A., & Umar, A. (2011). Microbial Features of Solid State Fermentation and Its Applications-An Overview: *Research in Biotechnology*, 2(*6*), 21-26.

Subramaniyam, R., & Vimala, R. (2012). Solid State and Submerged Fermentation for the Production of Bioactive Substances: A Comparative Study: *International Journal of Science and Nature*, 3(*3*), 480-486.

YOUR KNOWLEDGE HAS VALUE

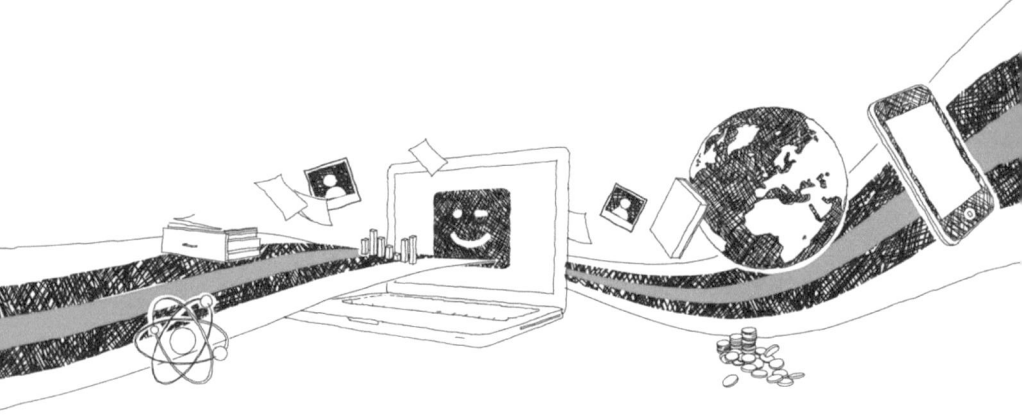

- We will publish your bachelor's and master's thesis, essays and papers

- Your own eBook and book - sold worldwide in all relevant shops

- Earn money with each sale

Upload your text at www.GRIN.com
and publish for free

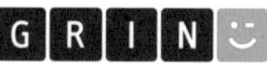